Neuroplasticity: Your Brain's Superpower

"In *Neuroplasticity: Your Brain's Superpower,* Dr. Douyon provides an elegant and encouraging summary of how the brain can heal itself. This book will be a useful resource for patients, caregivers, and providers."

—**JEREMY YVES CHARLES, MD**
Attending Physiatrist
Board-certified in Physical Medicine and Rehabilitation
Board-certified in Brain Injury Medicine

"Dr. Douyon presents novel ideas and new insights regarding the human brain and its workings in his book *Neuroplasticity: Your Brain's Superpower.* In his book he debunks old myths about the human brain and provides exciting new ideas. This book sheds new light on the wonderful nature of our brain and provides ideas on molding thought processes to overcome obstacles. Whether you are someone who has been personally affected by a neurologic condition or someone keen to understand the unparalleled potential of the human brain, this book would be a superb read!"

—**SISIRA YADALA, MD**
Neurologist/Epileptologist

"Finally, we have an expert in the field of neuroscience and neurology, who breaks down complex concepts and demystifies the workings of the brain, while putting the power back in our hands. Through his thoughts and reflections on neuroplasticity and neuroinfluences, Dr. Douyon, a physician and neurologist, unlocks the true power of the brain to help us heal and reach our full potential. If anyone wants to understand the secret behind the brain—our brain—and behind any forms of healing, this book is for you. Read it and share with your loved ones."

—**MARDOCHE SIDOR, MD**
Quadruple board-certified Psychiatrist
Author of *Journey to Empowerment* and
Discovering Your Worth

"*Neuroplasticity: Your Brain's Superpower*...provides a primer on brain structure and function in an accessible reader-friendly manner...consistent with an ever-expanding body of research attesting to the benefits of exercise and mindfulness and related forms of mental/brain training, Dr. Douyon reveals how these mind-body therapies work to foster neuroplasticity, preventively and for rehabilitation (providing hope for those who have been stricken by debilitating brain disease). Of special interest in this era of political unrest is a chapter on neurology of decision making, information processing and control and how cognition can play a central role in major societal events. This is a book that everyone should read, especially people who have always wondered about the brain and its mysteries. Dr. Douyon helps demystify the brain and neurological disorders; it provides hope and a way to exert influence over how one's brain can be protected as well as healed."

—**ROLAND A. CARLSTEDT, PhD**
McLean Hospital, Harvard Medical School
Integrative Psychological Services of New York City
American Board of Sport Psychology

"Neuroplasticity–I was briefly introduced to this term in medical school and then began to understand it during my rehabilitation training as I watched patients recover from different types of brain injuries. From a public perspective, neuroplasticity is a poorly understood and a rarely mentioned term, yet it is such a huge part of life. Dr. Douyon does an amazing job in his book of breaking down a complicated concept so we can understand how this term applies to many aspects of our life as he walks us through the Neuroverse."

—JAMES F. WYSS, MD, PT
Assistant Attending Physiatrist
Assistant Professor of Rehabilitation Medicine,
New York-Presbyterian Hospital

"In his book *Neuroplasticity: Your Brain's Superpower*, Dr. Douyon explores the emerging science of neuroplasticity in relation to common neurological disorders. The book is written in an easy to comprehend language and shall appeal to the casual reader looking to enhance and harness the healing power of the brain as well as to the neuroscientists among us."

—NITIN K. SETHI, MD, MBBS, FAAN
Associate Professor of Neurology,
New York-Presbyterian Hospital
Weill Cornell Medical Center, New York, NY

IZZARD INK PUBLISHING COMPANY
PO Box 522251
Salt Lake City, Utah 84152
www.izzardink.com

LIBRARY OF CONGRESS CONTROL NUMBER: 2019935014

Designed by Alissa Rose Theodor
Cover Design by Susan Olinksy
Cover Image: Garry Killian/Shutterstock
Interior Images: Christina Wheeler

First Edition April 23, 2019

Contact the author at info@theinlebrainfitinstitute.com

Paperback ISBN: 978-1-64228-100-2

eBook ISBN: 978-1-64228-101-9

Neuroplasticity

YOUR BRAIN'S SUPERPOWER

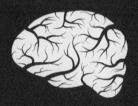

CHANGE YOUR BRAIN AND CHANGE YOUR LIFE

PHILIPPE DOUYON, MD

IZZARD INK
PUBLISHING

To Elias and Ismael
My greatest creations!

Contents

Preface

Imagine that suddenly you experience a strange feeling that you have never felt before or maybe you have felt it, but never gave it much thought. This time the feeling is different, more intense, but yet illusory, nearly immaterial, and at the same time uncontrollable. This feeling is causing you to descend into darkness and your next memory is of waking up in a hospital bruised, bleeding, in pain, and barely able to speak because your tongue has been badly bitten. Imagine your confusion. Imagine the sense of terror your loved one must have felt when he/she witnessed your first seizure and thought that they were helplessly watching your death before their very eyes. Imagine how your life would change when the doctor tells you that you have epilepsy.

How devastating it must be to be diagnosed with a neurological disorder? In an instant the life that we once knew dramatically changes. Without warning our central nervous system begins to fail us, our brains betray us, and our lives begin to deteriorate. Sometimes slowly, at times quickly, but always with devastating consequences, neurological disorders take captive our mental faculties and our physical bodies. They steal our memories, rob us of our identities, and distort our perceptions. Neurological disorders impair our abilities, weaken our extremities, deform our physiques, and cause physical and psychological pain. Medications hardly if ever undo the underlying cause of the disorder destroying our lives. At best, they may ameliorate some of the symptoms. With no way of changing our circumstances we are left powerless, at times hopeless, and desperately searching for some semblance of control.

What if we are not as helpless as we thought? What if our neurological health is within our control? It used to be thought that we lived with the brains and all its neurons and connections that we were born with. We used to think that our neuroverse™, all the existing cells and connections in our brains, only changed with the degeneration of disease and the degradation of old age. We used to think that we could only lose neurons and their connections. We now know differently. We know that our brains are influenced by everything around us, some of which are negative neuroinfluences™ and lead to the death and destruction of nerve cells and others which are positive neuroinfluences™ and cause the birth of new neurons and the sprouting of new connections. We know that our brains are capable of undergoing a tremendous amount of change throughout one's life. We also know that the power to implement those changes lies within us.

The brain's ability to change is called neuro-plasticity. Gathered here in one place is a series of thoughts about neuroplasticity, the ways in which the brain reacts and adapts to the things which influence its evolution, how that impacts our thinking, its applicability to different neurological disorders, and how the power to shape its destiny lies in the thoughts we contemplate and the actions we take. This book tries to present a more empowering view about the relationship we can have with our brains so that we can prevent its dysfunction and heal its injuries.

Neuroplasticity and The Human Neuroverse™

Nature shows us that life evolves, and has new and fantastic ways of adapting to its environment. For example, camels concentrate body fat in their humps instead of throughout their bodies which allows them to survive the desert heat. Life develops new senses, new organs, and new designs to cope with all the different stimuli influencing its existence. Our largest organ, our human skin, its color variable throughout the world, is a wonderful adaptation to protect us from the different exposures to ultraviolet radiation from the sun. The human brain isn't any different in its incredible ability to adapt to differing stimuli. Welcome to the wonderful world of Neuroplasticity.

In order to understand Neuroplasticity, we must first understand the structure of the brain. Its folded surfaces, its dense layers of neurons and supporting cells, and the vast networks within the cerebral hemispheres are what allow our brains to evolve with every experience and thought we have.

Grossly, the human brain is a three pound mass of a mixture of fat and water, pinkish beige in color. Its surface is characterized by long ridges and deep grooves, giving the brain more surface area, allowing the skull to encase more matter and information than it could muster otherwise. On the surface runs numerous arteries penetrating the brain at various locations, supplying the necessary blood and nutrients the brain needs to carry out all of its functions. Macroscopically, the human brain is divided into three distinct structures, the cerebrum, the cerebellum, and the brainstem, all of which can be further subdivided into various structures and functions.

The cerebrum, the largest part of the brain, evolved most recently in terms of our evolutionary history. Its midline is divided by a chasm that splits the cortex into right and left hemispheres, and grooves further carve the cerebrum into four distinct lobes. The cerebrum contains numerous substructures with their functions impacting everything from consciousness to creativity. Making up more than two thirds of the mass of the brain, it is the part of our nervous system responsible for critical thought, voluntary movement, communication, our sense of self and the world, and our ability to process and interpret information.

Lying beneath the cerebral hemispheres, in the posterior regions of the skull, is the cerebellum. With the numerous folia wrinkling its surface and the tree like pattern that decorates its anatomy, the cerebellum plays a role in cognitive functions such as attention and language, as well as equilibrium. However, the cerebellum is best understood for the role it plays in motor control. It doesn't initiate movement but it aides in the coordination and precision of movement. The cerebellum receives information from the brain and spinal cord, integrates that information to provide smooth, coordinated, and accurate movement. The cerebellum brings finesse to the motor system.

The cerebellum is attached to the brainstem by three distinct bundles of fibers that allows for the flow of information between these two structures. The brainstem is evolutionarily the oldest part of our brain. It is composed of three different parts, the midbrain, the medulla, and the pons. The brainstem is the connection between the brain and the rest of the body, as all motor and sensory fibers course through it. It also provides basic life functions, playing a vital role in cardiac and respiratory activity.

Despite the complex gross anatomy, it is the microscopic world of the human brain that gives it its reputation as being the most complex structure in the known universe. In fact, the brain and all of its components, is a universe within itself, which we will refer to as the Neuroverse™. The brain consists of over one hundred billion neurons and at least the same number of supporting cells, known as glial cells. Each neuron can have thousands of connections, often forming relationships with other neurons in regions of the brain widely separated, creating a vast and intricate cerebral network. Electrical impulses travel through this network at great speeds, like a jolt of electricity, allowing various neurons and individual networks to communicate with each other. The constant bursts of electrical activity twinkles like the stars in the night sky illuminating the matrix of the human brain.

Every component of the brain, every cell, receptor, and particle that makes up the Neuroverse™ erupted from stem cells within the embryonic structure that gives rise to the central nervous system. These stem cells differentiate into various neurons, those that specialize in discerning information from our senses, interneurons which receive and send information to other nerve cells, and motor neurons which send information to the muscles and glands of the body. All of these neurons migrate from their birthplace, expanding the fabric of gray matter that helps make up the anatomy of the human brain. As the neurons mature they develop trunk like axons to send information and branch like dendrites to receive information from other nerve cells. In between each axon and the neuron that it influences, a synaptic gap develops that allows them to communicate with each other through the spread of chemical transmitters that create an electrical current. The synapse is the point of communication between neurons. It is the space where information is communicated, processed, and integrated into the network of the Neuroverse™. In the human brain, a single neuron can receive information from tens of thousands of synapses, creating an intricate network of neurons, axons, and dendrites.

As the brain develops, it loses its uniformity. Neurons migrate and some begin to concentrate in great numbers near the surface of the brain. The density of nerve cells causes the brain to fold in on itself, giving it its characteristic appearance, and increasing the surface area. Neurons form with and with out long axons allowing for information to be disseminated across variable distances of the Neuroverse™. Principal neurons consist of long axons, acting like an expressway, conducting information over long distances, from one region of the brain to another. They allow for communication to take place over the vast space of the human brain. Local circuit neurons lack axons and exert their influence in the region in which their cell bodies and dendrites are located. There, they integrate and modulate information allowing us to process data from our internal and external environment.

Neurons are not the only cells to make up the Neuroverse™, in fact the microscopic brain is held together and supported by a constellation of cells called glial cells. The glial cells occupy the space in between neurons, outnumbering them, and performing functions to sustain neuronal health. They direct the migration of neurons during their development and produce chemicals that regulate the growth of axons and dendrites. Radial cells function as scaffolding, allowing immature neurons to migrate to their final destination. Astrocytes, named for its star like shape, provide structural support for neurons, helping to hold them in place. They help regulate the flow of ions and other chemicals in the synaptic gaps and help to repair damaged neurons following an injury to the brain. Microglia remove dead cells from the brain and help to protect the brain by directing immune responses and regulating inflammation. Oligodendrocytes insulate axons, allowing for information to travel faster from the body of the neuron to it's target nerve cell. Ependymal cells are responsible for the creation and circulation of cerebral spinal fluid, and make up the blood-CSF barrier. The glial cells function to protect neurons, hold them in place, insulate their axons, regulate the immune response, and remove dead cells. Glial cells help to regulate the metabolic activities of the Neuroverse™, keeping our brains fit enough to engage in the structural and functional changes that they need to evolve.

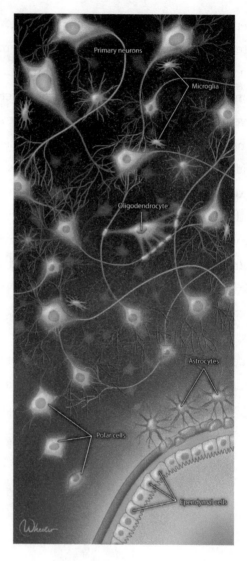

Figure 1: The Neuroverse - illustrating depicting the neurons, axons, dendrites, and glial cells within the brain. Neuroscientist, V.S. Ramachandran once said,".....the number of brain states exceeds the number of elementary particles in the known universe."

We used to think of the Neuroverse™ as fixed, and assumed that we were limited to the number of cells we are born with. But our view of the brain has shifted with the phenomenon of neuroplasticity. No longer do we think of the brain as static, not evolving, without the capacity to develop new neurons and make new connections. We now know that our brains have the power to create, and that we have this gift at our disposal throughout our entire lives. Our Neuroverse™ is capable of creating new neurons and building new connections, strengthening old ones, and pruning those nerve cells we no longer use.

The brain changes with everything that we experience. We know now that the Neuroverse™ is a dynamic place, influenced by every thought we have, every challenge we face, every new perspective we hear, and every habit we create.

In fact, the Neuroverse™ is capable of *tremendous* change. Every time we decide to learn something, we create new nerve cells and facilitate the creation of new networks. We don't *notice* the bursts of new neurons being formed or the creation of new synapses. For all the wonders that it can perform, the human brain is fairly naïve about its own inner workings. However, the evidence for neuroplasticity is tremendous and its impact is all around us.

The Neuroverse™ is influenced positively and or negatively by all of its surroundings: everything we encounter and think up. The Neuroverse™ is constantly evolving, making new networks, creating new neurons, and growing more connections. The Neuroverse™ is a dynamic place where nerve cells are reaching out to each other, disposing pockets of roving neurochemicals that find their way through the synaptic cleft to stimulate the ends of other nerve cells, communicating with and influencing their neighbors' actions. Whether neurons are born together or firing together with the same purpose in mind, they connect with each other through their dendrites and axons, creating fantastic networks of information and influence.

Neuroplasticity has an enormous impact on our brains' microscopic universe and in our lives. The Neuroverse™ and all the matter and exuberance contained within it not only reflects the microscopic framework of our brains, but also who we are as individuals and a society. Our collective brains right now are trying to tackle the global issue of climate change, potentially reinventing who we are as a society. Because of this, neuroplasticity's effect on the Neuroverse™ emphasizes our unlimited potential – not only as individuals, but humanity overall. This book's purpose is to demonstrate how neuroplasticity can impact every aspect of our lives - - including our neurological health, who we are as individuals, and how we evolve as a society.

Neuroplasticity is the phenomenon of how the brain is influenced and continuously changes with every experience that it encounters. Neuroplasticity is about the dynamics of our brains, about how our brains ebb and flow with every physical activity, positive or negative thought, and rousing emotional stimulus. It is the process of how our brains' structure changes in response to *every experience* we have. And it's about how these experiences cause neurons to be born or silenced, new neuronal connections to be made and old ones weakened, and about how much protection and sustenance is offered by the supporting cells to the neurons.

Neuroplasticity tells us about how we learn, evolve, regress, and recuperate from neurologic injury. It teaches us how we can grow into the individual we've always dreamed of being, and why we become stuck in self sabotaging patterns. Understanding neuroplasticity means that we can begin to understand the process of reaching our full neurological potential, learn how to minimize the risks of neurological disease, and heal the injured brain.

Our brains are different from other organs in our body. The heart is a pump that circulates blood and nutrients to support and sustain the body, especially the brain. The liver filters blood coming from the digestive tract, metabolizes drugs, and rids the body of chemicals and toxins, allowing the body and brain to function optimally. The kidneys filter blood ridding the body of wastes that would otherwise bring dysfunction to the brain. In some way, all of our other organs serve to protect the brain.

This is because the brain is *majestic*. It is the part of us that is strikingly similar to the universe, that connects us to a higher power, even to God. Neuroplasticity teaches us that our brains are so much more than an organ that receives input, interprets information, stores experiences, and sends out electrical impulses. It shows us that our brains are capable of creation, and allows us to be master of our neurological destiny, creator of our lives.

Neurons: The Framework of Neuroplasticity

Neurons are simply cells within our nervous system. Of all the cells in our body, they are the most remarkable, because they are uniquely shaped to receive and share information. They have specialized parts called axons to send information and dendrites to receive information. Neurons sprout dozens of extensions from their bodies looking for partners, or other neurons to connect to. Typically, one axon arises from each neuron and is responsible for influencing the activity of other nerve cells, while multiple branches of dendrites arise from body of the neuron to receive guidance and inspiration. The tree-like structure of these cells is designed to receive information, process it, and then send information to other neurons. This creates extensive networks of over one hundred trillion connections.

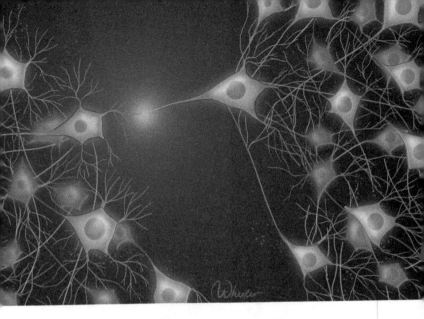

Figure 2: The human brain as a network – illustration of the human brain as an intricate network, consisting of billions of neurons and trillions of connections.

Despite the brain's more than 100 billion neurons, ninety percent of the cells within the cerebral hemispheres are not neurons at all, but supporting *glial cells* that sustain the neuron. These cells supply nutrients, rid the the brain of bacteria and viruses, remove dead cells, and hold the neurons in place, creating a framework that supports the web of information within our brains.

Why devote an army of glial cells to support neurons? Because neurons are where we process information. They are the source of our connection to the universe and to each other. It is in these networks where lightning strikes -- that neurons communicate and bond with each other by sending and receiving electrical impulses.

And neurons truly *do* radiate electrical energy. This energy is the spark that gives us the ability to learn, evolve, and change our brains. The energy that rests within each neuron fluctuates with the impulses that it receives from the other nerve cells it is connected to. The connection is a functional one, not literal. The synaptic cleft is the gap that lies between neurons where each cell is able to release the chemicals the cause bursts of electrical activity in its neighboring cell. Every thought and every action causes a burst of electrical activity among neurons, especially those in the same network that have been previously involved in similar thoughts and acts.

At the cellular level, neuroplasticity is about creating new connections between nerve cells and strengthening or weakening old ones. A new action or a new thought will recruit neurons into a new network, causing them to fire together in a new pattern. Repeating those thoughts or actions will stimulate that network of nerve cells more and more, reinforcing it and turning those ideas and activities into habits. *Not* reinforcing that group of neurons ✗ and all its connections will weaken the thoughts and behaviors that belongs to that network.

Every cell in our nervous system knows that the ✗ ability to evolve, the power to create, and the beauty of life is about connection and disconnection. Our brain's ability to be plastic comes from our neurons connecting, disconnecting, increasing and decreasing the strength of each link at every moment. No neuron lives in isolation, because isolation would surely mean death. Neurons survive and thrive due to the impulses that they receive from each other.

Every action that we take, thought that we have, dream that we dream; every emotion that we experience, person that we love, and individual who we care about is due to the connection that a group of neurons has. The majesty of life and the gift of neuroplasticity comes from the interplay of the network of neurons and their ability to share, communicate, and connect to each other.

The Ways In Which The Brain Changes Itself

There is always more than one way to do something in life, which neuroplasticity shows by offering several strategies to change the brain's structure and function. This amazing process occurs on a spectrum from our normal maturation to actions undertaken by the brain to heal a devastating neurological injury.

Remarkably, the ways in which the brain changes itself are not necessarily automatic, involuntary activities. Our actions play a significant role in neuroplasticity. Through awareness and understanding of the methods of neuroplasticity, we can actually establish a new relationship with our brains. We are not passive bystanders or potential causalities of a neurological injury. Instead, we can be active players controlling our brain's evolution, using them the way we wish, instead of letting our brains use us.

To become the leaders that our brains need, let's first look at some of the ways in which the structure and function of our brains change naturally throughout the course of life.

Neurogenesis, the birth of new neurons, is one of the critical ways in which the brain changes its structure. Until recently, it was thought that the adult brain was not capable of producing new neurons. People believed that the lack of stem cells within our brains meant that neurogenesis only occurred during the development of the embryo. This widely held maxim maintained that we were born with a fixed number of nerve cells and that injured or dead neurons could not be replaced.

However, Science now shows us that what we thought to be an incontrovertible truth turned out to be dead wrong. Neurogenesis not only extends beyond the embryonic period; it occurs throughout life. Synaptogenesis, the formation of new connections between nerve cells, takes places continuously, with every experience we encounter and thought we have. What's most remarkable is that lifestyle choices such as exercise can promote the birth of new neurons and the formation of new networks.

It's not just lifestyle choices that affects the structure and function of our brains. Our brains respond to cues they receive from their environment – both cellular and macroscopic worlds – in a process called developmental neuroplasticity.

This is a naturally occurring phenomenon that arises early in life, involving the rapid increase in number of nerve cells and the prolific spread of dendrites and axons to allow the baby to receive and tend to all the stimuli it will encounter. These neurons will then finetune their connections in conjunction with the environmental stimuli that they face. If they don't encounter the appropriate stimulus, these connections will be weakened and maybe lost so that the brain can devote resources to networks of neurons that it uses regularly.

When a neuronal network has been damaged, another pre-existing network of neurons can often reorganize itself to help compensate for the functions lost by the injury. This is called compensatory masquerade. This gives us alternative ways to perform the same functions. For example, some people may have an intuitive sense of direction, making them efficient at getting around from place to place. However, a brain injury may cause them to lose this spatial intuition; so going forward, they use landmarks to navigate their environment. The recognition of landmarks was a network that already existed, but is one they're now using differently to compensate for the deficit resulting from the brain injury.

Cross model reassignment occurs when an area of the brain deprived of its main stimulus develops different functions in response to new sources of inspiration. An example is someone who is born blind. In sighted people, the occipital lobe of the brain in response to light is primarily responsible for vision. In blind people, the occipital lobe – inspired by the sense of touch – changes its function to allow people to interpret the world around them through physical contact. This is why the blind are able to read braille.

Imagine the surface of the brain as a map. Each area represents one function or stores one particular type of information. When we carry out a behavior frequently or continuously reinforce information, the part of the map responsible for this strengthens and grows. For example, when learning a musical instrument, the areas of the brain responsible for participating in the process of playing grow with each practice. This is referred to as cortical remapping or map expansion.

Neuroplasticity offers us a variety of ways to shape our brains, evolve, and rebuild or compensate for neurologic and cognitive functions impaired by brain injury. In this way, it gives us hope that no matter the state of our brains, we can change for the better through a choice of different strategies. Our awareness of the process of neuroplasticity allows us to adapt to our circumstances, creating new and incredible lives for ourselves.

Neuroplasticity and Neuroinfluence™

We know by now that the brain is dynamic; it adapts to every thought we have, every action we take, and every experience we encounter. We also know that while these changes are microscopic – occurring at the level of neurons and synapses – the results are palpable. Not only do these adaptations lead to structural changes in the brain; they result in be-havioral differences, new perspectives, a shift in opinions, the developments of new skills, and the ability to heal old deficits.

The brain's ability to change indicates just how much its structure and function is shaped by ex-ternal and internal stimuli. The ability to affect the evolution, anatomy and physiology of the brain – as well as to dictate its progress or regression – is called Neuroinfluence™.

Neuroinfluence™ describes everything that im-pacts our brains' development. It concerns all the things that promote the birth or death of neurons, that cause new neuronal connections to develop and old ones to perish. It refers to those things that encourage synapses to form, neurotransmitters to be released, neurons to fire and wire together, and causes connections to strengthen or weaken. Neuroinfluence™ describes everything that our brains have ever and will ever come in contact with and the effect they have on neuroplasticity.

The brain responds to all stimuli by either giving birth to new neurons (neurogenesis), creating new connections (synaptogenesis), strengthening or weakening the networks which already exist, eliminating synapses (synaptic pruning), or pruning nerve cells. Everything that the brain encounters has the potential to shape its future. Therefore, everything is a neuroinfluence™, sculpting the brain either positively or negatively and in various degrees.

A positive neuroinfluence (PNI)™ is anything that promotes neurogenesis and synaptogenesis — any stimuli that creates new neurons and builds new networks. PNI™ helps the brain evolve, and results in the acquisition of knowledge or a new skill. The subject matter of the information learned does not contribute to the positivity or negativity of a neuroinfluence™. All that matters is that it causes the creation of new neurons and the expansion of the neural network. In fact, the content the brain takes in can be morally vile, lead to prejudiced thoughts and behaviors, tarnish a person's character, and negatively impact a community; but if it enhances the individual's neural network, it is still a *positive* neuroinfluence (PNI)™. Listening to new ideas whether good or bad, reading, thinking about things in a new way, developing new skills, exercising, and living a healthy lifestyle are all positive neuroinfluences™. A positive neuroinfluence (PNI)™ only refers to things that have a constructive impact on the development of our brains, regardless of how it manifests outwardly to our communities.

On the other end of the spectrum, a negative neuroinfluence (NNI)™ is anything that impairs or destroys neurons and synapses – something that has a negative impact on our brains' structure and function. Negative neuroinfluence (NNI)™ can include exposure to toxins such as drugs or alcohol. Traumatic brain injuries, concussions, degenerative brain disease, sedentary lifestyle, stress, and psychological traumas are all forms of negative neuroinfluences (NNI)™.

Every day, we are exposed to a whole host of stimuli that influence our brains in positive and negative ways. Our exposure to these positive and negative neuroinfluences™ helps to keep our brains dynamic. Who we are as individuals is partially based on this balance of positive and negative neuroinfluences™ in our lives. Therefore, to have control over how our brains develop, we need to be aware of the neuroinfluences™ shaping its evolution. Being cognizant of what is a neuroinfluence™, whether it has a positive or negative effect, and how that impacts the structure and function of our brains allows us to be in control of our own evolution.

Neuroplasticity and Stroke

There is no phenomenon that brings change to the brain's structure and function faster than a stroke. A stroke is the sudden cessation of blood flow to a specific region of the brain. It manifests as an abrupt, un-expected loss of our ability to move, communicate, and/or interact with the world around us. A stroke changes the reality of one's life in a split second. We experience the world drastically differently, our view of our own life is altered, and our body betrays us. In a sudden disabling attack, we are no longer who we thought we were. A stroke negatively influ-ences our minds, brains, and bodies all at once. It does so by causing neurons to die and the networks that they've created to perish, resulting in irrevers-ible neurologic damage.

Neuronal networks are irreversibly damaged when they don't receive enough blood flow from the vessels that supply them. The arteries that supply the different regions of the brain are tubes of blood carrying high concentrations of the oxygen and nutrients that neurons need to live. To obstruct this flow or decrease the amount of blood that bathes the brain negatively influences neuronal integrity and function. The severity of the obstruction and the length of time that it persists dictates the extent of the damage.

The death of neurons occurs quickly in response to this disruption of blood flow. After just a few minutes of being deprived of nutrients, the structure of the neuronal bodies in that region change. Millions of nerve cells at the core of the stroke begin to swell, rupturing their membranes, spilling their inner contents into the surrounding brain tissue. The resulting inflammation irritates neighboring neurons and puts pressure on nearby structures. Neurons in the areas surrounding the center of the stroke shrink in size, distorting their structure. Those neurons have yet to die, but they do become functionally impaired. As millions of neurons at the heart of a stroke die, billions of dendrites and synapses perish, destroying countless networks and damaging the entire brain network system.

When strokes are assessed on CT scans or MRIs, we see them as isolated areas of brain damage. Those images – which show the localized regions of the brain the stroke has affected as well as the networks of neurons that inhabit them – provide some factors on which a person's prognosis is based. The expectation is that the stroke victim's deficits will correlate with the function that we know that part of the brain is responsible for. However, neuronal networks are not confined to any particular area; they are widely distributed. Therefore, if someone has a stroke in an area of the brain responsible for the movement of their left leg, they may also experience other deficits.

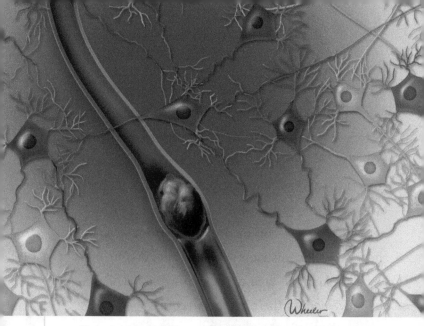

Figure 3: Neuroplasticity and Stroke - Illustration showing how the network of neurons, axons, and dendrites are damaged during a stroke. As a clot blocks the flow of blood to a specific area of the brain; damage to one area indirectly affects the entire network.

Imagine the entire brain as a huge, complex network of billions of neurons and trillions of connections, firing countless electrical impulses in every direction of the grid. Every function that the brain is responsible for is either directly or indirectly linked to each other. Therefore, a stroke that weakens *any* aspect of the link will hinder the networks of many brain functions.

A stroke can be a devastating event in the life of a loved one – or in our own lives. But neuroplasticity provides some hope here. Even when strokes destroy and damage neuronal networks, we can use neuroplasticity to birth new neurons, rebuild lost connections, and reorganize surviving networks and synapses. Our brains are capable of a tremendous amount of healing, particularly through conscious effort. The brain is wiring and rewiring at every opportunity.

Often when a person is left disabled by a stroke, they compensate by primarily using their stronger parts and ignoring their disability (i.e., using a right arm if their left arm has been disabled.) However, failing to use the weakened or paralyzed body part teaches the brain that it no longer needs to invest in a neuronal network for that function. The remaining neurons and synapses that would have compensated for those cells lost begin to deteriorate.

To regain function after a stroke, people need to consciously and continuously work on what they've lost. It can be a difficult process; but doing so will prompt nerve cells neighboring the stroke to sprout new dendrites into the damaged part of the brain – and can recoup some of the lost functions. Neurogenesis and synaptogenesis take place, helping to rebuild the damaged network and retrieve what was lost. Re-teaching the brain what used to come so easy and learning new tasks can of course feel cumbersome and even frustrating. However, it's incredibly important, because it helps to rewire the entire whole brain network system – remodeling the brain and helping people reclaim their lives.

Neuroplasticity and Epilepsy

There is no other neurological event that exemplifies the malfunction of neural networks or circuits more explicitly than a seizure. In normal brain function, neurons communicate with each other through the spread of chemical transmitters, which creates an electric current. A seizure occurs when the current becomes faulty. This results in a burst of electrical activity in the brain, similar to a short circuit. As a result, when a seizure occurs — at times without warning — we can lose control of our brains, our consciousness, and our bodies. A seizure negatively influences the brain by locking neurons in an electrical storm, hijacking our neural networks and our lives.

The excessive neuronal electrical activity that results in a seizure causes a transient, episodic event that changes our behavior, alters the way we perceive our environment, and can even eliminate our ability to control our movements. Epilepsy is defined as having recurrent unprovoked seizures or having an increased risk of having periodic events. Simply, we can divide epilepsy into two big categories: those with seizures that originate from one particular part of the brain or focus are diagnosed with *focal epilepsy*. People whose seizures are due to a burst of electrical activity involving the entire brain from the very beginning of the episode are diagnosed with generalized epilepsy.

A seizure can occur as a result of many things. It is a symptom of something negatively influencing nerve cells, their connections, and the networks they associate with. When the structure of the brain has been warped by a tumor, damaged by a stroke or trauma, or irritated by a bleed within the brain, the risk of a seizure increases. When neurons' function has been impaired by toxins such as alcohol or drugs, poisoned by wastes that a dysfunctional liver or kidney is unable to excrete, or affected by altered levels of electrolytes, a seizure is more likely to occur. In this way, a seizure is an expression of malady and injury to the neurons. It is their cry for help. As a result, any chance of healing must take a look at relieving the offending cause.

A seizure is not just the result of an assault on our neural networks. Recurrent seizures also have a negative impact on the wiring within our brains, priming the brain to *continue* to short circuit. While we may not be able to predict how seizures spread across neural networks, we know that they do. And we know that this in turn increases the potential that other areas of the brain will become a focus from which seizures may originate.

A seizure beginning in one area of the brain affects millions of neurons at the onset, and involves countless more as the seizure spreads across different regions. Envision the brain's huge, complex network of billions of neurons and trillions of connections, firing countless electrical impulses in every direction. Now imagine the impact on the brain's entire neural network when these millions of neurons, their axons, and dendrites are suddenly seized by a surge of electrical activity. Every function in which those neurons play a role – directly or indirectly – and every individual network that they associate with are impaired by the seizure.

Once seizures become chronic, it is more difficult to treat epilepsy. Neuronal networks strengthen in chronic conditions, misfiring neurons have more frequent bursts of electrical activity in patients with medically refractory epilepsy, and poorly functioning neurons deteriorate over time. In fact, recurrent seizures not only effect the composition and function of nerve cells; they also cause structural changes in the brain. In some people with uncontrolled epilepsy, parts of the brain undergo atrophy; that is, they begin shrinking due to this repeated excessive stimulation. These seizure-induced neuroplastic changes increase epilepsy's progressive nature of in some people.

Seizure induced-neuroplasticity doesn't just shrink the brain; it can also add to the existing neural networks. New nerve cells can be created after a seizure. These new neurons migrate to the areas of neuronal injury after a seizure occurs and integrate themselves into the neural network. Sometimes, these immature nerve cells connect to the network or migrate to the wrong areas of the brain, possibly aggravating the seizure disorder.

However, this same process underlines the amazing potential of neuroplasticity to heal the brains of people with epilepsy. If we could promote neurogenesis and support the migration of mature neurons to the areas within the brain prone to abnormal burst of electrical activity, then we could encourage healing to take place at both the microscopic and gross structural level. We could stimulate neurogenesis and synaptogenesis to rebuild the damaged network, helping to repair what is injured, and regain control of our brains, our bodies, and our lives.

Neuroplasticity and Parkinson's Disease

Famous actor Michael J Fox once said of living with Parkinson's Disease, "With Parkinson's, it's like you're living in the middle of the street and you're stuck there in cement shoes and you know a bus is coming at you." And of course, there's nothing you can do. But with neuroplasticity – is there?

Parkinson's Disease is an illness that commandeers a person's mind and movement, leaving them cognitively impaired, stiff, slow, tremulous, and frozen in a state of unbridled neurological deterioration. It is caused by the degeneration of the brain. Specifically, Parkinson's Disease occurs as a result of the degradation and death of neurons, especially in the part of the neuroverse™ called the substantia nigra. An area in the middle of the brain stained black because of its richness in the pigment melanin, the substantia nigra is made up of neurons which contain the chemical dopamine. Dopamine is a necessary component for normal movement; it is a positive neuroinfluence™ on the parts of the brain that play a central role in our motor control.

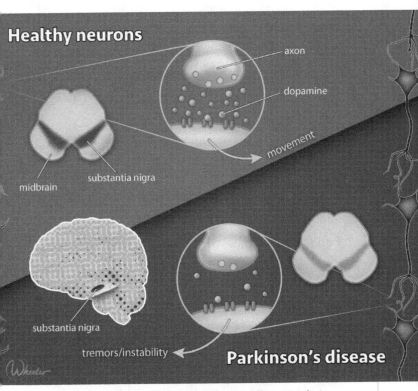

Figure 4: Neuroplasticity and Parkinson's Disease - illustration depicting a healthy neuron receiving an adequate amount of dopamine and below that a neuron in Parkinson's Disease being deprived of adequate amounts of dopamine. The substantia nigra is a structure in the midbrain, stained dark by the neuromelanin found in dopamine rich neurons. Death of neurons in the substantia nigra is associated with Parkinson's Disease.

To date, the main treatments for Parkinson's disease have been to boost the amount of dopamine in the brain and ease the deficits that result due to a lack of dopaminergic neurons. Dopamine is a neurotransmitter that effects many aspects of our lives. It is a chemical that gets released from neurons to influence other nerve cells, modulating our executive functions in the frontal lobe and influencing our mental state. It alters the white matter fibers that control our movements, impacts the hormones released by the pituitary gland, and controls the reinforcement and reward system that drives our motivations – and therefore our behaviors. Compared to other chemicals in the neuroverse™, our brains don't make a lot of dopamine; but this chemical's influence is widespread and powerful. To lose some of the dopaminergic neurons can have a devastating impact, resulting in the symptoms associated with Parkinson's Disease, especially impairments in movement.

Our brains develop so that we can move, explore our environment, travel to new domains, have fresh experiences, learn, and evolve. Because it is a neurodegenerative disorder that impairs movement, Parkinson's disease is a negative neuroinfluence™ on our entire brain. As people with Parkinson's become less mobile, they learn less and take in less new information. The neuroplastic brain has less opportunities to create new neurons, build new networks, and reinforce old connections in the immobile person. As a result, nerve cells wither, the neural network begins to break down, and the brain atrophies.

The resulting cerebral atrophy seen with Parkinson's Disease is likely the result of a few factors: the lack of dopamine nourishing the brain pathways it influences, and the lack of stimulation that occurs with immobility. People with Parkinson's Disease develop impairments in thinking, memory, attention, concentration, and perception at higher rates than those without Parkinson's. These cognitive deficits can lead to dementia – making Parkinson's the second most common neurodegenerative disorder behind Alzheimer's Disease.

If Parkinson's Disease is the result of the loss of neurons that specialize in secreting the neurotransmitter dopamine, then our neuroplastic brain's potential to create new neurons can be an ally in managing Parkinson's. Our brains have the remarkable potential to learn, create, wire, and rewire the neural network. People whose mobility have been restricted by a neurological disorder such as Parkinson's disease tend to do the same thing that stroke victims do; that is, they'll often avoid the area with which they struggle, which is what needs the most attention. Failing to work on the movements that have been impaired by the loss of dopamine causes further damage to our neural networks. By being conscious of our bodies and training the brain to move them in ways that may offset the deficits, we can stimulate the birth of new neurons and create new pathways through which nerve cells can communicate.

In fact, the growth of the neural network not only occurs throughout the entire brain, but in areas primarily affected by Parkinson's Disease. Engaging in behaviors that protect against losing dopaminergic neurons and that promote neurogenesis and synaptogenesis can help slow disease progression and improve the quality of our lives.

Neuroplasticity and
Multiple Sclerosis

There are a number of offenses that can injure our neuronal networks by attacking nerve cells and the trillions of connections that exist within the neuroverse™. In addition to some scenarios we've already covered such as strokes, seizures, and neurodegenerative disease, these assaults on our brains can occur with the abnormal growth of cells seen with a tumor, or a traumatic head injury whose impact wave rips axons and dendrites from their neurons, tearing the network apart. However, with multiple sclerosis (MS), the human body's very own immune system attacks the gray matter (neurons) and white matter (axons), damaging our brains, and leading to significant neurological disability.

Multiple sclerosis occurs when instead of protecting the body against foreign invaders, our immune system's cells attack *myelin*, the sheath of fat that wraps around the axons of our neurons. Myelin insulates the projections of our nerve cells, increasing the speed that the electrical signal travels from one neuron to the next. The result of this attack on myelin is that the wave of electrical energy across neurons slows, disrupting the ability of parts of our neuroverse™ to communicate and causing significant neurologic impairment. Our immune system can attack myelin anywhere in the brain and spinal cord, resulting in a whole host of potential symptoms. With repeated attacks, the myelin sheath and the axon below it becomes irreversibly damaged and scarred, and permanent neurological deficits take hold.

Multiple sclerosis also destroys *oligodendrocytes*, the cells responsible for creating and maintaining myelin. As the disease progresses, extensive demyelination of various regions of the central nervous system occurs. Axons begin to break down, neurons are unable to communicate efficiently if at all, and a propagation of symptoms (that vary based on the regions of the brain and spinal cord affected) takes hold. People can suffer the pangs of losing the strength in their muscle while watching their bodies atrophy. They can develop numbness and tingling in their extremities, develop a painful loss of vision, and lose control of their bowels and bladder. The disease can rob people of their ability to express themselves and or their ability to explore the world around them without the help of a gait aide.

The symptoms of multiple sclerosis are not just the result of demyelination. The other negative neuroninfluence™ at play in this disease process is inflammation. The attack on myelin by the immune system triggers a release of inflammatory cells that can do more damage to neurons, their axons, dendrites, and synapses. The corresponding swelling which occurs can potentially decrease the flow of electric current between nerve cells. Inflammatory cells may further promote demyelination, and trigger the loss of axons and neurons, further disrupting the neuronal circuit.

Multiple sclerosis damages the neuroplastic brain by causing myelin sheaths to fail, damaging axons, and forming scar tissue. It impairs neurons' ability to communicate by altering their ability to fire electrical impulses efficiently. MS does not just affect the areas blemished by a scar or flooded by inflammatory cells; it hinders the entire brain's neural circuit. The damaged nerve cells underneath the scar negatively impact on all the neurons to which they're connected. Therefore, to treat multiple sclerosis, those afflicted must take care to heal the entire neuronal network, modifying and correcting how neurons fire.

Healing a brain impaired by MS starts by repealing the demyelination and inflammation injuring neurons and their connections. Removing these offending processes helps to restore balance to the brain, decreasing the abnormal firing of neurons. Taking away the pressures that stress the neural network can help to alleviate MS symptoms. Once demyelination and inflammation are relieved, it's paramount to make lifestyle modifications that promote neurogenesis and synaptogenesis. Creating new neurons, forming new axons insulated by myelin, and growing new connections can increase the efficiency and strength of electrical impulses travelling between nerve cells. Rewiring the neural network can allow those afflicted with multiple sclerosis to lead better lives.

Most people have felt anxiety at some point in their lives. It is a normal every day occurrence that can be triggered by public speaking or taking a plane ride. Anxiety is a physiological response that occurs when we are faced with a danger that threatens our lives, when we perceive possible danger, or even when we are uncertain of the outcome of something import- *ruminate* ant to us . Anxiety involves feelings of nervousness, worry, uneasiness, and at times intense fear. It encompasses elevations in our heart rates; taking short, quick breaths that are difficult to control; profusely sweating; chest pains; and even the sense of impending doom.

We've all experienced anxiety, because it is part of our normal response to stress that originates in our brains, which directly influences other aspects of our bodies. The hypothalamus, located on the underside of the frontal aspect of the brain, is charged with managing our response to stress by influencing the release of certain hormones.

Its connection to the pituitary, a pea sized gland at the base of the brain, and the adrenal glands, which sit on top of our kidneys, play a role in managing our anxiety.

A baseline amount of anxiety is normal. It helps focus our attention and determine whether we need to meet our threat head on or flee for safety. Anxiety only becomes a disorder when the hypothalamic pituitary-adrenal network becomes hyper-excitable. This can throw us into a state of excessive worry and nervousness – despite the fact that no threat is present. As a result, we begin to respond to normal situations as if they were threatening, worrying ourselves to the point where we can not function normally.

The hypothalamus is part of a network of neurons constituting the limbic system, which plays an important role in emotion and memory. People with anxiety disorders feel fear due to the *memory* of danger – whether that memory is true or the misinterpretation of a previous experience. Once that fear memory has been wired in, it is reinforced with every bout of anxiety. Like all other parts of the brain, the hypothalamus is plastic, capable of change both in structure and function.

Emotions such as anxiety are powerful promoters of neuroplasticity. The more we focus on our anxieties and respond in an anxious way, the worse our state of uneasiness and apprehension gets; the more sensitive the hypothalamic pituitary-adrenal network becomes, strengthening the circuit of fear that handicaps us. By constantly thinking of those things which make us nervous, the more deeply we ingrain the circuit of anxiety.

The treatment of anxiety disorders is intimately tied to the use of medications that manipulate neurochemicals or minimize the physical symptoms produced by an anxious state, such as increased heart rate, elevated blood pressures, chest pain, or shortness of breath. These medications attempt to stabilize physiological responses to stress so that we don't overreact to everyday situations. However, they often don't eliminate the underlying problem; and they certainly don't alter the circuit of anxiety in a way that normalizes the function of our stress response.

The dysfunction of the neural circuits of anxiety are often learned. We learn to fear non-threatening things or react in an anxious way to everyday situations based on experiences we have had in our past.

With each anxious response, we make that anxious circuit even stronger. The first law of neuroplasticity is, *"Neurons that fire together wire together."* In other words: the more we respond in a fearful way to a given situation, the stronger we insulate that neural circuit. The second law of neuroplasticity is, *"Neurons that fire apart wire apart."* So, repeatedly *inhibiting* the anxious response to a given situation can break the circuit – and help relieve our anxiety.

Healing the anxious brain means interrupting the connection between the worrying thoughts and the stress response. If we're able to keep the body calm when facing anxiety-provoking situations, our neural networks are less likely to be hyper-excitable and the brain is less likely to worry. Also, concentrating on something other than the worry when encountering circumstances that cause uneasiness can help grow new neuronal circuits. The new circuit will compete with the old dysfunctional one, thereby weakening it, promoting a healthier response to stress, and improving the quality of our lives.

Neuroplasticity and Depression

Depression is a significant cause of disability and morbidity, resulting in tremendous suffering in the lives of many people. It can occur in isolation or in association with multiple medical, psychiatric, and neurological disorders, and can even mimic other diseases. In fact, depression can present with such debilitating impairments in memory, learning, perception, understanding, and the consolidation of information that it's symptoms can fool doctors into thinking that their patients have dementia. The varied appearances of depression can make it difficult to recognize, difficult to diagnose, and therefore difficult to treat.

The diverse symptoms that depression can cause are not arbitrary manifestations of a sad state of mind. Instead, they are signs of the structural and microscopic changes that take place in the brains of depressed individuals. Neuroimaging studies show that major depressive disorder is associated with decreased volume in areas of the brain crucial to memory, emotional stability, the ability to learn new information, motivation, decision making capabilities, sleep, sex, eating, and the stress response. These changes in the hippocampus, the amygdala, the frontal lobe, the prefrontal cortex, the hypothalamus, and other regions of the brain are *measurable*, and have been calculated to be as high as a fifteen percent reduction in these areas. When altered, these interconnected structures form a circuit of depression, decreasing the brain's ability to react and adapt appropriately to various stressors.

Whether mild or severe, depression is much more than just a feeling of sadness. It is an unshakeable sense of hopelessness and helplessness that results in an indifferent approach to all aspects of life. Depression leads to a feeling of social disconnection – a detachment from society that's intimately connected to the breakdown of the neural circuitry that occurs in the depressed brain.

The structural changes in the brain associated with depression are at least in part due to the release of chemicals that are a negative neuroinfluence™. Stress changes our brains. In particular, the release of the stress hormone cortisol – over a long period of time or in high quantities – kills neurons, especially in the hippocampus, which is the center of emotion, memory, and the autonomic nervous system. Cortisol binds to receptors in the hippocampus, helping us to create memories and learn new information. However, too much cortisol damages the network of nerve cells within the hippocampus. It causes axons and dendrites to break down, retract from neighboring neurons, and significantly changes the circuitry. Excess cortisol prevents neurogenesis and synaptogenesis from taking place. In addition to impairing areas of the brain like the hippocampus, it also prevents those regions from rewiring and healing themselves.

Without the ability to heal itself, the depressed brain becomes locked in a state of gloom and despair. Its neural circuitry breaks down, neurons are unable to communicate with each other, and the brain loses its ability to adapt. The neural network is designed to allow neurons to share and transmit information through the release of neurochemicals across synapses. As a result of the physical changes that take places in the brain's micro-circuitry – including the degradation of axons and dendrites and the loss of neurons – these neurotransmitters are unable to exert their influence.

Nerve cell connection, nerve cell growth, and the overall function of the neural network plays a significant role in depression. This is why, among all the antidepressant treatments, electroconvulsive therapy – or ECT – has the highest response rates and gives people with depression one of the best chances of recovery. ECT is a brain stimulation procedure in which electric currents are intentionally passed through the brain, triggering a seizure.

ECT does much more than just shock the brain out of the darkness of depression back to the light. It goes beyond allowing a stuck network of nerve cells the opportunity to reset itself. Electroconvulsive therapy is a spark of creation. It boosts the release of brain-derived neurotropic factor, a neurotransmitter that plays a vital role in neuroplasticity and neurogenesis. Electroconvulsive therapy encourages the creation of new neurons and promotes the connection of nerve cells. It does this in the hippocampus, a significant player in the depression circuit, and an area of the brain responsible for memory and emotions.

Treating depression – whether through ECT, medication, and therapy, or a combination of these – prompts new pathways to form in the brain, undoing the aberrant circuits that lead to the sense of helpless resignation. Healing depression changes the brain's micro-circuitry, which in turn relieves the physical effects of depression and improves how people feel about themselves.

The goals of depression treatment are to achieve remission, return people to optimal levels of psychosocial functioning, prevent the relapse of depression, and minimize adverse effects from treatment. However, neuroimaging studies show that after treating an acute episode of depression, the decreased volume and activity of some of the brain regions in the depression circuit normalizes. Seeing depression as a problem in the neural circuitry allows one the ability to make the necessary changes to the brain to undo depression, allowing people to reconnect to themselves and society, and live more fulfilling and happier lives.

Neuroplasticity and Addiction

Addiction is a brain disorder that affects tens of millions of Americans. It is a chronic disease that takes control of one's brain, changes its circuitry, and makes that person dependent on the object of their compulsion – whether it's a substance like alcohol or drugs, or an activity like gambling, or even shopping. Addiction plays on those circuits which link reward, motivation, and memory, thereby influencing our biology, our social interactions, our spiritual wellbeing, and our psychological health. It changes who we are in a fundamental way, enslaving us to the pathological pursuit of detrimental substances and behaviors in order to relieve a craving, and/or search for the good and reinforcing feeling of reward.

Drug addiction interferes with the normal functioning of our neurons. Drugs like marijuana bind to receptors within our brains, causing the release of chemicals which alter how our neurons work. Other dugs like cocaine stimulate neurons to release huge amounts of the neurotransmitter dopamine and prevent the body from breaking it down, which makes us feel good and motivates us to continue to seek out that feeling from the drug. Drugs change not only the functioning of our neurons but also their connections making it easier for us to use and reuse those drugs, leading to addiction.

We don't need drugs to cause surges in dopamine levels that cause addiction. Excessive gambling and shopping can also change our brains by boosting dopamine, motivating us to pursue the rush that some of us feel when engaging in those behaviors.

Like many other chronic diseases, addiction is progressive. It's always interfering with the quality of our lives, and causing significant pain and morbidity. It sets us on a destructive path that usually leads to premature death. When the object of our dependence is suddenly withheld – that is, when we can't access the thing or behavior we're addicted to – physical signs take hold. Addiction is characterized by withdrawal symptoms such as disturbances in mood, changes in appetite, changes in sleep pattern, shaking, and headaches.

✗   However, the physical symptoms of withdrawal don't have the most significant impact. It is the psychological withdrawal symptoms, such as cravings and anxiety, that often drive relapse. Addiction usually involves cycles of relapse and remission, as efforts to cut out the obsessions from one's life are unsuccessful. In addition to this physiological reliance, addicts often have remarkable behavioral problems. Their addiction can cause them to engage in criminal activity or lead to impaired motivation and cognitive dysfunction – thereby compromising interpersonal relationships and diminishing the role of the important things in life, such as family, and friends.

✗   So – what is the source of this distraction, that causes our brains to turn away from important people and things, and focus instead on addictions? The answer is *dopamine*, the neurotransmitter that promotes reward seeking behavior, brings us pleasure, and triggers addiction. Addictive substances and behaviors takes control of the dopamine system in our brains. In particular, they increase dopamine in a part of our brains called the nucleus accumbens, which plays a vital role in motivation, reward, pleasure, and reinforcement learning. All the things that people become addicted to such – work, alcohol, nicotine, caffeine, food, drugs, sex, gambling, video games, shopping, risk taking behaviors, even seemingly positive activities like running – boost dopamine in the nucleus accumbens. Regardless of whether the outcome of this dependence is the accumulation of store bought items, a drug induced high, or winning races, all addiction boosts dopamine in the nucleus accumbens, the reward center of the brain.

Drugs are one of the most powerful addictive substances. Illicit drug use can cause dopamine levels to soar as high as 800 percent beyond their normal levels in the nucleus accumbens. This dopamine release prompts a significant amount of pleasure without requiring much work. It also makes that thing which triggered the release of dopamine to stand out amongst all other stimuli. This, in turn, forces our brains to pay attention to it, heightens its level of importance, and increases our motivation to seek it and its reward out at all costs.

In addition to giving us pleasure, dopamine surging through the nucleus promotes neuroplasticity – something we know permanently changes the brain. This ability to change the brain's structure is what makes addiction such a difficult disorder to treat. Addiction is a negative neuroinfluence™; it changes the connections in our brains in a way that causes us to develop automatic dysfunctional responses to external triggers. Once the brain has focused in on that which triggered the release of dopamine, the prefrontal cortex stimulates the hippocampus to remember everything there is about the substance or behavior which led to that wonderful feeling of reward. We learn everything about the scenario in detail, creating new nerve cells, sprouting connections with every association we make. Every time we think about our addiction, make new associations, relive it, and experience it, we flood our brains with more dopamine, which further increases the synaptic connections, wiring them in even stronger. We build an intricate neural network dedicated to our addictions, with an arrangement of grossly obvious associations and indirect connections serving as triggers for an automatic maladaptive response.

Addiction does more than spur on the creation of new axons, dendrites, and synapses. Changes occur within the *neurons themselves* that promote the pursuit of these substances and behaviors.

DeltaFosB is a protein that accumulates in neurons within our nucleus accumbens when we exhibit addictive behaviors, such as abusing drugs and compulsive running. Each time the we respond in a maladaptive way or ingest that substance, we accumulate more DeltaFosB in our neurons. This protein lingers in our system long after we've stopped taking the drug or performing the actions to which we are addicted. The long lasting presence of DeltaFosB suggests that it can change the genes within our neurons, damaging our dopamine system. In fact, studies show that when our brains contain neurons with higher levels of DeltaFosB, we develop sensitivity, requiring less drugs or maladaptive behavior to crave it intensely. Therefore, we *want* more and more of the substances and behaviors that relieve the cravings, and reflexively act in a way to do anything to get our rewards.

When we're forced to go without the substances and behaviors we crave, our addicted brain begin to show all the signs of dependency. Without the flood of dopamine that our brains have become accustomed to, the brain activates the stress response of the hypothalamic pituitary-adrenal network previously discussed in the section on anxiety.

Our bodies will begin to withdraw. We develop irritability, restlessness, and anxiety. The heart begins to race, blood pressure soars, and our bodies begins to tremor and twitch uncontrollably. The sudden drop in dopamine leaves our brains depressed and anxious. Even long after we've stopped the using addictive substance or engaging in the activity, our brains remain in a delicate state in which normal daily stressors are enough to awaken the cravings of addiction.

This makes the treatment of addiction is a long process. It begins with minimizing the symptoms of withdrawal caused by the irritability of the hypothalamic pituitary-adrenal network, and boosting dopamine in an organic and healthy way. It then continues with building new neural networks. Because neuroplasticity is competitive – that is, new neurons and synapses will form at the expense of old ones we no longer use – we need to build new networks that will free us from the pathological pursuit of the substances and behaviors that control our addicted brains.

Neuroplasticity and Memory

Our memories define us. They make our lives recognizably different from that of everyone else. Memories give our lives meaning. By storing and processing every experience we've ever had, we have a reference point to which we can compare every new encounter. Memory allows us to learn – not just about the procedure of doing things or for the successful completion of an examination, but about ourselves as well.

Memory keeps track of the story of our lives. That is why the prospect of of getting Alzheimer's disease is so terrifying, or why we panic when we begin to notice small lapses in memory. This idea that we will lose ourselves, forget who we are, and what we've meant to our families, friends and communities, frightens us.

For everything that memory represents, memory is about *connection* as far as our brains are concerned. It is about the impact of the connection amongst neurons and the strength of those networks. Memory is the epitome of the amazing sensitivity, power, and complexity of neuronal connection. It helps create our sense of reality. By sending and receiving electrical impulses to each other and connecting with each other, neurons allow us to store information, learn, create, and reminisce about our lives.

If memory is about neuronal connections and the strength of those networks, then memory impairment arises from disconnection. This can occur when neurons don't connect in ways we would like them to, or because some process weakened the web of preexisting connecting nerve cells. There is a wide range of neuropathologies that can cause memory dysfunction by affecting our memory systems' neural networks. In fact, anything associated with structural changes in the brain (i.e., stroke, tumors, Alzheimer's Disease) or any toxic or metabolic issues that damages neurons and their networks (i.e., drugs, alcohol, liver dysfunction) can cause memory impairment.

Structural changes, toxic exposures, and metabolic derangements aren't the only forces that cause memory impairment. We often allow *ourselves* to negatively impact our own memory systems.

Our society has become so distracted lately that we don't give our neurons a chance to receive information, encode and process it, and than consolidate the information. Yet we still expect our memories to retrieve something that we never gave our brains a chance to learn.

Our phones, social media, the television, family and friends, and even our own thoughts engross us so much that sometimes, what we assume is memory loss is simply due to a lack of registering information. We weren't able to register information, because we lacked of focus and attention. In short, we don't give our neurons a chance to make new connections and wire them in nowadays.

Another negative influence on our memory networks is our tendency to avoid learning new information. Most people feel comfortable with what they already know. They therefore surround themselves with people who think like they do. We participate in the same activities (the ones we know best); we travel familiar routes; and we read articles that support our ideological beliefs. We reinforce the networks we already have instead of making new neurons, new connections, and building new networks.

Once again, let's imagine memory as a complex web of nerve cells radiating with energy, firing and misfiring billions of electrical impulses every second from every interconnecting point of the network. This is the case, then we can envision an imperfect system where mistakes occur from time to time. Occasionally, it will take more time than we would like to remember something, or we may have instances where our memories fail us. It's completely normal for such a complex system to not work perfectly every single moment.

However, our *response* to this imperfect system is what matters most. If we focus anxiously on every memory lapse and tell ourselves that our memory is bad, then we create that network of failure and reinforce a message of a poor memory. If we expect that our memories will begin to fade as we age, then that is the message we give our brains. We set up our memories and life up for failure.

We can improve our memory by promoting neuroplasticity and remembering that no matter how old we get, our brains are capable of learning throughout our entire lives. The ability to acquire new skills and knowledge is a gift that we need to take advantage of. Not only does it lead to a more fulfilling life; it also helps to avoid the degeneration of our brains and aids in healing injured neural networks. By exposing ourselves to new experiences and learning new skills (i.e., like new languages, taking up new hobbies, learning to play a musical instrument), we can create new neurons with new axons and dendrites, and build new neural networks. This is how we enhance our memory. And if we allow ourselves to learn new things with passion and emotion, then our memory will be that much stronger. Emotions are the most powerful way to wire in a memory. Regardless of whether the emotion has a negative or positive influence on our brain, once added to a memory, it wires it in, cements it, and sews that memory into the fabric that defines our lives.

Neuroplasticity and
The 2016 Presidential Election

There is no denying that the 2016 Presidential election was a contentious one. Each party was able to mobilize its supporters, creating a fierce base of impassioned loyalists willing to overlook actions and comments that may have been arguably unbefitting of an American President. The vitriol and violence associated with this election has caused a divide in our country, going so far as to ruin friendships, strain families – even cause a plethora of "unfriending" throughout social media.

Some argue that politics is not personal; it's about a love of country, the support of a particular platform, and the general direction in which you want to see the country move. But this election became *very* personal, for a lot of people. It left millions of individuals questioning the morals and values of the country, their neighbors, their families, and their friends.

But what if the Presidential Election had nothing to do with morals and values, campaign platforms, or love of country? What if it was all in our heads? What if it's based on how we are programmed as individuals and communities? What if it results from how our brains are wired, the kind of neuronal networks we've created?

As we know by now: our brains record everything we've ever been told, every thought that's crossed our minds, every lesson we've ever been taught, and every encounter we've had. When exposed to information, our brain takes it in and compares it to *every neural network* that already exists within it. If it is completely new data, the brain stores it, and it becomes the foundation for the development of a new network at a later time, given the right amount of repetition. If it's information to which we've already been exposed, the brain wires it in to preexisting networks, strengthening those pathways. It becomes a program, automatically controlling our thoughts and actions. The more we're exposed to similar information, the stronger the program gets. Regardless of whether they are based on facts, the programs become our truths, our perceptions. And we therefore base our actions and voting patterns on them.

Politicians need our votes. They know that in order to get them, they need to get in our heads and program us. Politicians need to influence us and at times, that requires altering our perceptions to match their political platforms. This is how they get us to vote for them: by drilling into our heads what they think are the country's biggest issues.

So, if some of our brains had already begun laying down pathways in line with the messages a particular candidate was communicating – based on our own personal experiences and our own thoughts – then that person has our vote. Every time we listen to their speeches, read their words in newspapers or online, and listen to the media analyze every sentence he or she has uttered, it reinforces and strengthens our neural pathways. This merges our truth with their ideas. If you live in Chicago, and have witnessed the violence or lost friends and family to death by guns, then it likely resonated with you when President Donald Trump says things like, "The American carnage stops right here and stops right now." You may be able to relate to the idea of "American Carnage" because it reinforces the program of violence that your brain has already created. If you were personally affected by the tragic shootings at Sandy Hook Elementary school in 2012 – or any other gun related violence – then you likely agreed when Secretary Hillary Clinton called for expanded background checks for guns and stricter gun control measures. Your brain had formed neuronal networks about gun violence, the dangers of guns, and the carnage that they can cause.

In this way, a politician's success is based on whether they can reinforce those things that our brains already know to be true. And if they can get us to *feel* something about those issues – then even better.

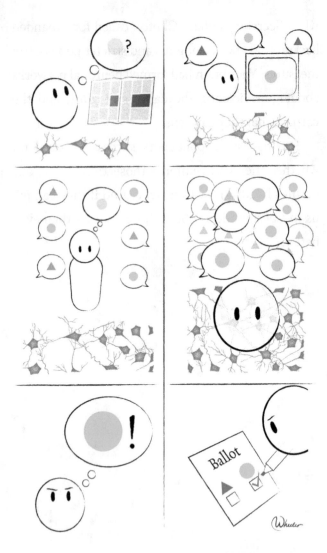

Figure 5: Neuroplasticity and the 2016 Presidential Election - cartoon showing the influence that repeated stimulation has in shaping our brains and neuronal networks, and the impact that has on the decisions we make at the ballots.

The issue of violence and particularly gun violence carries an emotional charge in this country, and politicians know that emotions are a key ingredient in getting our votes. They want us riled up, because emotions strengthen our neural networks. In fact, emotions are even more powerful than repetition when it comes to creating and fortifying our neural pathways. It's easier and quicker to connect with us and program us if what a politician is saying triggers a strong emotional response. That is why there are so many negative campaign ads, and why politicians make some ridiculous claims about their opponents. Think about the strong emotional impact of phrases like "Crooked Hillary Clinton" or "....because you'd be in jail." Odds are, these statements strongly reinforced neuronal pathways that had already been formed about an arguably corrupt Clinton career. Whether factual or not, it became the truth for millions of Americans. They believed it because their brains took in those messages, compared them to every neural network it had previously stored, and wired it in – thereby strengthening that program.

What we believe about ourselves, our lives, and our politics comes from the information we get from television, the internet, the newspaper, social media, our parents and other family members, our friends, our colleagues, religious leaders, and politicians. We form neural networks based on the information we receive from all of these sources, whether that information is true or not. How – sometimes, even *if* – we vote is based on how well campaigns are able to program their messages into our heads, creating and strengthening our neural networks, altering our perceptions, and shaping our realities. In a lot of ways, being an "informed" voter has less to do with the facts and more to do with how well politicians, their surrogates, their campaigns, and their political action committees manipulate our neural pathways. They know that we vote the way we are programmed to vote.

But there's good news: these programs are not necessarily fixed. As we know, our brains are always evolving, and neuroplasticity is constantly occurring. To establish new programs requires *awareness*. We must be cognizant of the information to which we are being exposed, and conscious that preexisting neural pathways have biased our thinking. Once we have insight into the way information influences our actions and thoughts, then the next step is to control the information we are taking in, leading our brains down the path we choose. It is only then that we can truly vote our conscience.

Neuroplasticity and Mindfulness

We know by now that neuroplasticity makes our brains capable of shaping us into the individuals we've always wanted to be. Thanks to this phenomenon, we're able to create the lives we've always envisioned for ourselves and our communities. This awesome creative power is within our control, but harnessing it requires awareness. We must be cognizant of all the things that influence the strength and connectivity of the cells within our brains. We must be conscious of the stimuli which promote neurogenesis and synaptogenesis so that we can continue to evolve. We must also remain knowledgeable about those noxious stimuli that cause injury and death to neurons – the things that inhibit our ability to control our neurological destiny. Influencing neuroplasticity requires one to be mindful of all the positive and negative things that impact the health and function of our brains.

Being mindful provides twofold benefits: it helps us remain aware of those things that influence our brains, while changing the structure and function of our brains by building new networks and reorganizing old ones. Mindfulness is a state of complete self-awareness, without distractions or judgment. It is about being *in the moment* with love and compassion, realizing the importance of the present and relating to it with peace and sympathy. Being mindful allows us to check in with ourselves and assess our moods, physical state, cognitive and emotional wellbeing.

Because it keeps us in the moment, mindfulness allows us to let go of the regrets of the past and the worry that tends to be associated with the future. By diminishing these stresses, the mindful brain is less susceptible to the toxic influence of stress related hormones and chemicals. This allows the brain to generate new neurons and build new networks. We see this occur in several areas of our brains, but particularly in those regions that allow us to reach a higher level of awareness.

Mindfulness is about establishing a heightened level of awareness of ourselves. When someone is mindful, one of the places we see changes in the brain's structure and function is where the temporal and parietal lobes meet. This region plays an important role in how we experience ourselves. The temporal parietal junction is responsible for processing and coordinating the information that our brains receive from our internal organs with the influences of our external environment. It attends to the information we get regarding our body's place in space. Injury to this area can therefore lead to an "out of body" experience.

The temporal parietal junction also plays a crucial role in our ability to connect and sympathize with others, helping us to recognize and understand their emotions. It is an important region for theory of mind, our ability to understand things from other people's perspectives, and therefore facilitates the compassion we have for each other. Being mindful increases the density of neurons and dendrites in the temporal parietal region, allowing us to be more aware of ourselves and those with whom we surround ourselves.

The ability to look within ourselves, be aware of any changes occurring within our internal and external environments, and determine the significance of these experiences is due to the activation of a region of our brain called the *posterior cingulate cortex*. The increase of nerve cells and connections in this area allows us to adapt our behaviors and perceptions to these changes.

On the other hand, an inability to adapt to new conditions can lead to significant mood disturbances. Neurotransmitters which regulate are moods are created in the brainstem. Areas located within our brainstems form new neurons and synaptic connections in response to mindfulness training. Modulating neurotransmitters have long been targeted by pharmaceutical companies for the treatment of depression and anxiety disorders. Yet mindfulness can impact these neurotransmitters in ways that pills cannot, boosting their production through neuroplasticity by creating new neurons.

The hippocampus is the part of the brain best known for its neuroplastic capabilities. It is an area of the brain critical to learning, memory, and emotional response. Mindfulness-based training has been shown to increase the nerve cells and synaptic connections in this region. The result has been improved memory and the ability to regulate one's emotional responses.

Being mindful allows us to be aware of the physical and the emotional changes occurring in our bodies and minds at any given moment. This focused attention allows us to take the time to check in on our mental, physical, and emotional well being. It encourages our brains to attend to what matters most to us in that moment, heal injured regions, and create new nerve cells and neuronal networks. Being mindful puts one on a path of awareness, compassion, creativity, leadership, and in direct command of neuroplasticity.

Neuroplasticity and Exercise

Our bodies have been engineered to move. We have hundreds of muscles, some of which give us power for explosive movements, while others enable feats of endurance. Our bones support our bodies and provide the framework that our physique needs for physical activity. Our joints, the place where two bones meet, add the flexibility that our skeletal system needs to maneuver. The combination of our muscles, bones, and joints creates a musculoskeletal system capable of walking, sprinting, jumping, pulling, pushing, lifting, squatting, dancing, and carrying out any form of exercise, movements that result in the expenditure of energy.

Our central nervous system is at the helm of our ability to exercise. Our brains and spinal cords are largely devoted to learning, planning, controlling, and executing our voluntary movements. The hundreds of billions of neurons and their trillion connections integrate the information we receive from all aspects of our physical world to manipulate our movements. The process is cyclical: our complex motor system does not just involve the brain's impact on movement, but also the influence that exercise has on shaping our brain's structure and function. Exercise is one of the most dominant manipulators of neuroplasticity, and is a powerful positive neuroinfluence (PNI)™.

Exercise exerts its influence on the brain in multiple ways. However, it's the direct impact that movement has on neurogenesis and synaptogenesis that makes it such a potent stimulator of neuroplasticity. Exercise causes the release of proteins – in particular, Brain Derived Neurotrophic Factor (BDNF) and Glial Derived Neurotrophic Factor (GDNF) – that build and maintain the structure of our neural networks. These factors promote the creation of new neurons; they cause nerve cells to sprout more axons and dendrites, increasing the possibility of their connections. They also allow neurons to communicate more efficiently with each other by insulating the connections they have and remodeling their synapses.

Exercise also triggers the release of other chemicals: Insulin Growth Factor 1 (IGF1), Vascular Endothelial Growth Factor (VEGF), and Fibroblasts

Growth Factor (FGF). All of these fuel learning by building and repairing damaged blood vessels. These factors work in concert strengthening and expanding our neural networks, decreasing our risks of cognitive decline and dementia.

Benefits of Exercise
on the Brain

Brain-derived neurotropic factor (BDNF)	Promote creation of new neurons
	Stimulate new axons & dendrites
Glial-derived neurotropic factor (GDNF)	Insulate and strengthen existing connections

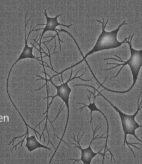

Insulin growth factor 1 (IGF-1)	Build new blood vessels (angiogenesis)
Vascular endothelial growth factor 1 (VEGF)	
Fibroblast growth factor (FGF)	Repair damaged vessels

strengthened neural networks

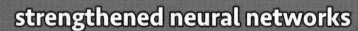

Figure 6: Neuroplasticity and Exercise - illustration depicting the influence exercise has on shaping the brain by providing substances that trigger the creation of new neurons, axons, and dendrites, as well as strengthening old neural connections. The chemicals released by engaging in exercise also minimize the risks of degeneration and stimulates healing in an injured brain.

Exercise is our fountain of youth. It not only keeps our bodies strong, but it also helps to offset the risk of the brain degeneration process as we age. Exercise becomes even more important as we approach middle age, and/or if we experience some insult to our brains. Its tremendous ability to create new neurons, enhance the connections we already have in our brains, and build more networks is something that nothing else we've discovered has the ability to do.

The creative and regenerative capabilities of exercise are just one element of its significance. The protective effect that exercise confers on the brain by reducing cardiovascular risk factors such as hypertension and diabetes is another tremendous benefit. This results in the brain being more freely bathed by the nutrients it needs to sustain all of its activities. Exercise promotes the health of our brain in ways that other modalities (i.e., medications) cannot, and with fewer risks of negative side effects.

To use our brains to their fullest potential, to witness the majesty of their creative powers, to enhance the healing capabilities of our neurons and synapses, exercise needs to be at the heart of any regimen designed to promote a healthy brain. To be sedentary will likely bring about an increased risk of damage to the structural integrity of our neural networks, without being readily able to stimulate the inherent healing processes within our brains. The clinical results are impaired neuronal functioning, difficulty learning, increased depression and dementia, and a diminished quality of life. Moving our bodies inspires our brains to create new neurons, build new connections, and grow our neural networks. Exercise helps stave off cognitive decline, promote lifelong learning, maintain and enjoy the relationships we have with our family and friends, appreciate the beauty that the world has to offer, and improve the quality of lives for longer.

Conclusion

One of this book's goals is to help establish a new under-standing of our brains and the relationships that we have with them. The aim is to show us that we are not passive pawns beholden to its sparks of creativity, the sluggishness of old age, or the dysfunction of disease. We are in the driver's seat of how our brains function. We have more control to shape the destiny of our brains than we ever thought. Our brains are constantly evolving – and *we* are the inspiration behind that evolution. They change with the messages that we give them. They adapt to fit our focus both in thought and behavior. We are the catalysts of neuroplasticity. It is a completely natural process that occurs from the time we are in our mother's womb and has the potential to continue until we take our last breath.

Our brains don't need to atrophy as we age. They have the potential to build, repair, and heal throughout our lives. We can create new neurons and synapses at any given moment. New neural networks are laid down and reinforced with every new material learned, subject studied, thought replayed, and movement repeated. The key is to keep our brains engaged and to lead them down a path where we are continuously acquiring new skills and strengthening old ones. A healthy brain is constantly learning, improving, and avoiding toxins like alcohol and drugs that could impair any aspect of the neuroverse™. It takes the time to be present in the moment, minimizing stress, and decreasing exposure to those things that negatively influence neurons and their connections, and impair the process of neuroplasticity.

Another motive of this book is to help change our perspective of neurological disorders. My hope is to show that these disorders occur as a result of damage to our neural networks and that that injury can have widespread neurological and psychological repercussions. This book is meant to ignite a conversation about expanding our treatment strategies to involve the principals of neuroplasticity in order to change the underlying pathology, heal the injury, and repair and regrow our neural networks. By targeting neuroplasticity as a treatment strategy for neurological disorders, we can evolve from a healthcare system which focuses on symptom management to one that can prevent and undo the damage done by any pathological process.

To take control of our neurological health and to change the relationship we have with our brains requires us to expand our perspective and understanding of how our brains work. Neuroplasticity offers us the opportunity to do just that. It provides a sense of empowerment, the ability to lead our brains down a path of optimal health, and gives us the ability to *control* our neurological destiny.

Glossary

Alzheimer's Disease: a progressive neurodegenerative disorder characterized by cognitive impairments included but not limited to the inability to learn new information, loss of memory, mood and behavioral changes, and language dysfunction. Alzheimer's disease is a type of dementia.

Anxiety: a normal temporary emotion in which people feel fear, worry, stress and develop physical symptoms such as increased heart rate in response to a stressor. Occasional anxiety is a normal part of life.

Anxiety Disorders: a group of mental disorders in which constant worry and fear can keep someone from carrying on with their everyday life. Anxiety disorders include panic disorder, specific phobias, social anxiety disorder, and generalized anxiety disorder.

Astrocytes: star shaped glial cells within the brain and spinal cord that have many functions including maintaining blood vessels and play a role in repair and scarring after an injury to the brain.

Axons: threadlike portion of the neuron that allows neurons to communicate with each other by carrying information from one neuron to another neuron.

Cerebellum: part of the brain at the back of the skull which plays an important role in motor control.

Cerebrum: large part of the brain that is divided into the left and right cerebral hemispheres.

Dementia: Refers to a broad category of progressive brain diseases that are characterized cognitive impairments, including but not limited to memory loss, emotional problems, difficulty with language, and behavioral changes.

Dendrites: threadlike portion of the neuron that allows neurons to communicate with each other by receiving information from other neurons.

Depression: Mood disorder characterized by persistent feelings of sadness and loss of interest.

Ependymal cells: cells which form the lining of the ventricles (fluid filled spaces) within the brain.

Epilepsy: a neurological disorder characterized by recurrent seizures.

Glial Cells: most abundant cell types in the brain and spinal cord whose various functions are to support neurons.

Hippocampus: a part of the brain located in the temporal lobes which plays an important role in memory formation.

Limbic System: a system of neurons and networks within the brain which helps control emotions.

Microglia: glial cells within the brain and spinal cord that are main form of defense.

Mindfulness: a state in which one is present in the moment without judgment.

Multiple Sclerosis: a chronic neurological disease in which there is damage to the myelin sheaths covering the nerve cells in the brain and spinal cord.

Myelin: the substance that surrounds the axons of neurons and increases the speed at which electrical activity travels.

Neurogenesis: the process by which new neurons are born.

Neuroinfluence™: the ability to effect the development, evolution, anatomy, and function of the brain and spinal cord.

Neurons: specialized cells within the nervous system which receives and sends electrical signals throughout the body.

Neuroplasticity: the ability of the brain to adapt, change, and form new neurons and new connections in response to learning and injury.

Neuroverse™: the brain and all of its components including but not limited to all of its neurons, connections, and supporting cells.

Oligodendrocytes: a glial cell which produces myelin.

Parkinson's Disease: degenerative brain disease which affects the neurons that make dopamine.

Radial Cells: cells responsible for producing all of the neurons in the brain.

Seizure: a sudden burst of electrical activity in the brain. It can cause temporary changes in behavior, movement, feeling, and consciousness.

Stroke: death of cells in the brain that occurs as a result of the sudden cessation or reduction of blood flow to that area of the brain.

Synaptic Cleft: the gap that lies in between adjacent neurons in which impulses pass by diffusion of neurotransmitter.

Synaptogenesis: the formation of synapses in between neurons.

References

Caldwell, DG. 2012. Intelligent Influence: The 4 steps of highly successful leaders and organizations. Intelligent Influence Publishing Group. 228pp.

Chopra, D., Tanzi, R. 2012. Super brain: Unleashing the explosive power of your mind to maximize health, happiness, and spiritual well-being. Three rivers press, New York. 320pp.

Chopra, D., Kafatos, M. You are the universe: Discovering your cosmic self and why it matters. Harmony Books, New York. 276pp.

Coyle, PK. 2016. Symptom Management and Lifestyle Modifications in Multiple Sclerosis. Continuum. 22: 815-836.

Doidge, N. 2007. The brain that changes itself: Stories of personal triumph from the frontiers of brain science. Penguin books, New York. 427pp.

Doidge, N. 2016. The brain's way of healing: Remarkable discoveries and recoveries from the frontiers of neuroplasticity. Penguin books, New York. 427pp.

Helmstetter, S. 2013. The power of neuroplasticity. Park avenue press, Florida. 278pp.

Hess, CW., Okun, MS. 2016. Diagnosing Parkinson Disease. Continuum. **22:** 1047-1063.

Kreiger, SC. 2016. New Approached to the Diagnosis, Clinical Course, and Goals of Therapy in Multiple Sclerosis and Related Disorders. Continuum. **22:** 723-729.

Matthews, BR. 2015. Memory Dysfunction. Continuum. **21:** 613-626.

Morgan, JC., Fox, SH. 2016. Treating the Motor Symptoms of Parkinson Disease. Continuum. **22:** 1064-1085.

Miyasaki JM. 2016. Treatment of Advances Parkinson Disease and Related Disorders. Continuum. **22:** 1104-1115.

Nair, DR. Management of Drug-Resistant Epilepsy. Continuum. **22**: 157-172.

Raine, A. 2013. The anatomy of violence: the biological roots of crime. Vintage books. 478pp.

Ramachandran, VS., Blakselee, S. 1998. Phantoms in the brain: probing the mysteries of the human mind. HarperCollins. 328pp.

Ratey, J. 2008. Spark: The revolutionary new science of exercise and the brain. Little, Brown and Company, New York. 294pp.

Sagan, C., Druyan, A. 1980. Cosmos. Ballantine books, New York. 432pp.

Schulz, PE. 2015. Depression. Continuum. **21:** 756-771.

Seifert, T. 2014. Exercise and Neurologic Disease. Continuum. **20:** 1667-1682.

Shah, AA., Han JY. Anxiety. Continuum. **21:** 772-782.

St. Louis, EK. Diagnosis of Epilepsy and Related Episodic Disorders. **22:** 15-37.

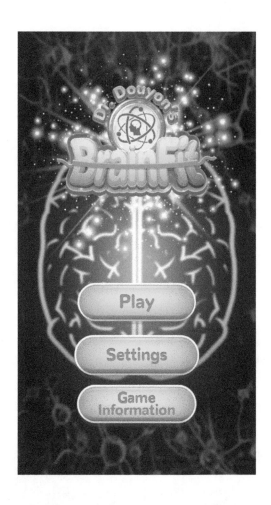

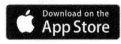 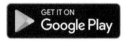

Creator: Philippe Douyon, MD
www.inlebrainfitinstitute.com

Developer: Burke Business Consulting Firm
www.bbcfirm.com

CPSIA information can be obtained
at www.ICGtesting.com
Printed in the USA
LVHW082032300720
661978LV00003B/33

9 781642 281002